HEALTH ISSUES

STEROIDS

Karla Fitzhugh

HODDER
Wayland

an imprint of Hodder Children's Books

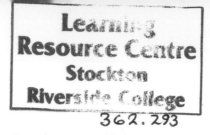
© 2003 White-Thomson Publishing Ltd

White-Thomson Publishing Ltd,
2-3 St Andrew's Place, Lewes,
East Sussex BN7 1UP

Published in Great Britain in 2003 by Hodder Wayland, an imprint of Hodder Children's Books.

This book was produced for White-Thomson Publishing Ltd by Ruth Nason.

Design: Carole Binding
Picture research: Glass Onion Pictures

British Library Cataloguing in Publication Data
Fitzhugh, Karla
    Steroids. - (Health Issues)
    1. Steroids - Juvenile literature 2. Steroids - Physiological aspects - Juvenile literature
    I. Title II. Nason, Ruth
    362.2'99

ISBN 0 7502 4376 7

Printed in Hong Kong by Wing King Tong

Hodder Children's Books
A division of Hodder Headline Limited
338 Euston Road, London NW1 3BH

Acknowledgements

The author and publishers thank the following for their permission to reproduce photographs and illustrations: Bridgeman Art Library: page 18 (Musee Municipal Antoine Vivenel, Compiegne, France); Corbis: cover and pages 1 (Tom & Dee Ann McCarthy), 4, 6 (Ariel Skelley), 11 (Dimitri Lundt), 15 (Paul Barton), 19 (Bettmann), 21 (Tom Stewart Photography), 23 (Julien Hirshowitz), 25 (ROB & SAS), 30 (Eric K. K. Yu), 31 (Jose Luis Pelaez), 33 (Michal Heron), 34 (John Henley Photography), 38 (Pete Saloutos), 39 (Roy Morsch), 41 (Randy Faris), 42 (Tom & Dee Ann McCarthy), 43 (James W. Porter), 44 (Lawrence Manning), 45 (Jose Luis Pelaez), 47 (John Henley Photography), 49, 50, 53 (Rick Gomez), 54 (Mug Shots), 57 (Russell Underwood); Angela Hampton Family Life Picture Library: pages 5, 8; Popperfoto: pages 14, 17, 20, 24; Science Photo Library: pages 10 (Dr P. Marazzi), 27 (St Mary's Hospital Medical School), 29 (Scott Camazine), 36 (Zephyr); Skjold Photographs: pages 13, 52. The illustrations on pages 9, 28, 32 and 59 are by Carole Binding. The illustrations on page 35 are by Michael Courtney.

Note: Photographs illustrating the case studies in this book were posed by models.

Every effort has been made to trace copyright holders. However, the publishers apologise for any unintentional omissions and would be pleased in such cases to add an acknowledgement in any future editions.

Contents

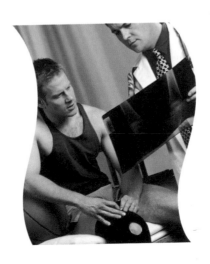

Introduction
Anabolic steroids

Anabolic steroids are a group of man-made drugs, which some people take for non-medical reasons. These people are usually hoping to increase the size of their muscles and lose some of their body fat. Often their aim is to increase their physical strength or achieve a look that they feel will appear 'healthy' and attractive.

The drugs are all similar to the male sex hormone testosterone, in the way that they act in the body. This is the hormone that moves into action particularly in males during puberty, bringing about growth and changes in the voice, skin and body hair. But people who use anabolic steroids take them in doses that are tens or even hundreds of times higher than natural hormone levels. Taking anabolic steroids for non-medical reasons is known as steroid abuse, and, like all drug abuse, it carries risks.

Steroids and sport
The pressure to win sometimes leads sportspeople to try taking anabolic steroids to boost their stamina and performance.

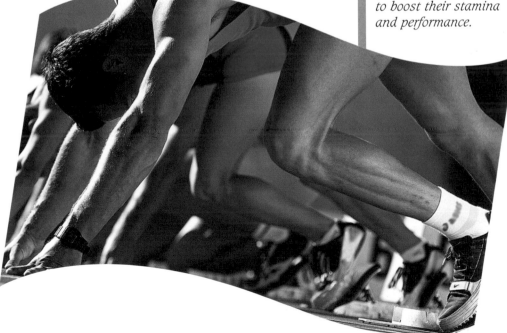

The real risks of steroids

The unwanted side effects of anabolic steroids range from mild and temporary to severe and permanent, and are especially bad in women and teenagers. Acne (spots) and greasy hair and skin are common. In about half of all anabolic steroid abusers, the drugs make the body retain water. This can lead to high blood pressure, putting the person at risk of heart disease and stroke. The drugs also raise the type of cholesterol in the blood that is linked to an increased chance of heart disease.

The side effects are most likely to be permanent in teenagers and women. In teens, anabolic steroids can cause seriously stunted growth, and there is no treatment for this condition. Women can suffer from permanent changes such as growth of beard and body hair, breast shrinkage and a deepening of the voice.

Many users report mood changes while they are on the drugs. Sometimes these are pleasant, but often users say they feel irritable or aggressive, and they may have difficulty sleeping. Depression is also a possibility, and some people say that the feelings of depression last for months after stopping taking the drugs.

Changes in mood, personality and behaviour can badly affect a person's ability to do their job, or their school or college work.

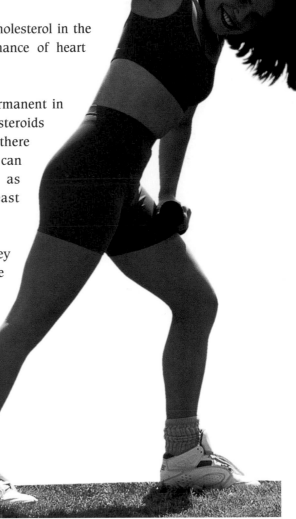

Building muscle

Many fitness regimes include using weights to strengthen muscles. But some people try to build their muscles more quickly by taking anabolic steroids.

They can also be damaging to friendships and family life. Users can sometimes find themselves on the wrong side of the law, depending on the legal status of anabolic steroids in the country they live in. Being caught taking anabolic steroids can also mean the loss of a job, sponsorship or sports scholarship.

Who takes them?

Doctors legally prescribe anabolic steroids for patients who have severe muscle wasting after illness or surgery, or for patients with severe anaemia who need to make more red blood cells. It was athletes who first took anabolic steroids for non-medical reasons. They thought that the drugs would make them more muscular and stronger, and able to recover faster from hard workouts. They were trying to give themselves an unfair advantage over other competitors, which most people would describe as cheating.

In more recent years, anabolic steroids have been used to boost physical appearance. Western society has become more and more concerned with the way people look, and there has been an increasing obsession with bodies that are very different to the average build, such as those of bodybuilders and supermodels. These unusual body types are often advertised to us as some kind of 'ideal way to be', although these people are often underweight or unhealthy in other ways.

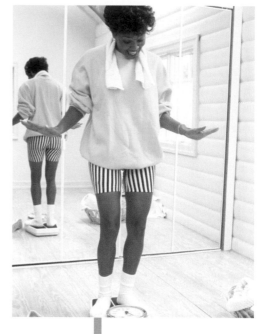

Body image
Some people base their sense of self-worth solely on weight or body shape.

Studies suggest that around half of all anabolic steroid abusers are teenagers, and half of this group take these drugs to change their appearance, rather than to boost their sporting performance. Anabolic steroids should never be looked on as a quick fix or an easy way to lose weight and tone up muscles. Taking these drugs will not have an effect on body shape unless a person is very fit and active already, and there are all the unwanted side effects to think about too.

What can be done?

Use of anabolic steroids was banned by the Olympic Games Committee in the 1970s, and there are official bodies all around the world that are responsible for drugs testing in sport. In some countries it is illegal to take anabolic steroids, and in other countries it is illegal to sell them without a doctor's prescription. Many of these laws are under review, and may become stricter.

There are other ways of making the drugs less attractive to users, such as educating people about the real dangers of anabolic steroids and helping them to find better ways to improve their body image and self-esteem. When some people insist on continuing to use anabolic steroids in spite of the risks, they can sometimes be persuaded to avoid the most dangerous behaviours, such as sharing dirty needles with other users.

About this book

Abusing anabolic steroids can harm health, relationships and careers. There are many different stories about how safe or how dangerous they are, and much of the information passed on between users is hearsay and has not been scientifically proven. This book aims to explain the real risks and effects of anabolic steroids.

'A friend who takes steroids says they're perfectly safe, but someone else told me I'd go mad or die of liver cancer if I ever tried them. I'm confused about the whole thing, and don't know who to believe.'
(Pete, aged 15)

Chapter 1 looks at what anabolic steroids are, and how they work in the human body. It also looks at the drugs that are most commonly abused, and the law. Chapter 2 examines the history of legal and illegal anabolic steroid use, and why some people are tempted to try these drugs. In Chapter 3, the true physical health risks of anabolic steroids are explored. Chapter 4 looks at the effects of steroid abuse on mental health, and Chapter 5 is for anyone who wants to give up steroids, or is worried about a friend or relative who might be taking these drugs. The Glossary on page 60 explains words that might be unfamiliar, and on page 62 there is a list of organizations that can be contacted for more help and information.

1 What are steroids?
Their actions on the body

Anabolic steroids are manufactured drugs that are identical to, or very similar to, testosterone in both their chemical structure and their action. Testosterone is the most powerful of several sex steroid hormones made in the human body. Looking at the actions of testosterone in the body helps us to understand the effects of anabolic steroids.

Testosterone

Testosterone is one of many different natural steroid hormones. All of them are made in the body from one basic building block, a fatty substance called cholesterol. They all have a similar structure: four rings of carbon atoms. What makes each type of hormone unique is the arrangement of other atoms that are attached to one of the carbon atoms (sometimes called the number 17 carbon atom). For each hormone, the attached atoms are a unique arrangement of carbon (C), hydrogen (H) or oxygen (O).

Teenage changes

When puberty begins, the hormone testosterone is released into the bloodstream, causing physical and emotional changes that turn children into adults.

What are hormones?

Hormones are chemical substances made naturally in special cells and glands around the body. They allow the body to fine-tune many different processes. Hormones are transported in the blood and act as chemical messengers, giving orders to the cells in certain tissues and making them act in a specific way. For example, in males, testosterone is produced by specialized cells in the testicles, and when it is carried via the bloodstream to skeletal muscle cells, it tells them to start building up more protein.

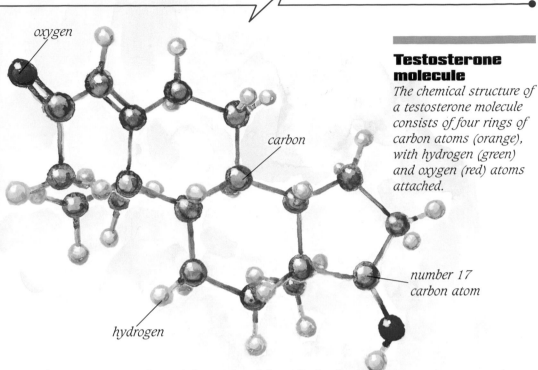

oxygen

carbon

number 17
carbon atom

hydrogen

*The chemical structure of
a testosterone molecule
consists of four rings of
carbon atoms (orange),
with hydrogen (green)
and oxygen (red) atoms
attached.*

In males, testosterone is mainly produced by cells in the
testicles, called the Leydig cells. It is released into the
bloodstream, which carries it to cells all around the body.
In both females and males, much smaller amounts of
testosterone are produced in other parts of the body such
as the adrenal glands, just above the kidneys.

For males and females, testosterone is essential for normal
growth, development and the functioning of the
reproductive organs. It also stimulates the growth of body
hair and the deepening of the voice in males at puberty.

How hormones give orders to cells

The cells within the tissues of our bodies have areas on their surfaces called receptor
sites. They are the perfect size and shape for particular molecules such as steroid
hormones to 'lock on to'. As a molecule binds to a receptor site, a 'chemical
message' is delivered, causing certain changes to the metabolism of the cell. For
example, when testosterone or anabolic steroid molecules bind to receptor sites on
the cells making up the oil glands in the skin, this stimulates the cells to produce oil
at a faster rate and the skin becomes more greasy than normal.

Anabolic and androgenic effects

Testosterone and anabolic steroids all have both anabolic and androgenic effects. Anabolic means 'building up'. Anabolic steroids stimulate the production of protein inside skeletal muscle cells, and this makes the muscles grow in size, when combined with exercise and a high-protein diet. Vigorous exercise is the starting point for all bodybuilding, because it naturally stimulates the muscles to grow, but lots of protein is needed for this process. It is thought that anabolic steroids make it easier for the body to retain protein, and so the muscles stay looking bigger for longer than in people who exercise but don't take the drugs.

The anabolic action of steroids may also increase muscle strength, although not all scientific studies agree on this. In addition, steroids seem to reduce the proportion of body fat. Testosterone and anabolic steroids can stimulate the growth of the long bones in the arms and legs, before and during puberty, and they can encourage the body to make more red blood cells.

The androgenic effects are the sexual changes that happen to males at puberty. Testosterone and anabolic steroids have a number of 'masculinizing' effects including: growth of body hair, growth of beard, tissue growth in the larynx (voice box), causing the voice to deepen or 'break', subtle changes to face shape, and coarsening of the skin.

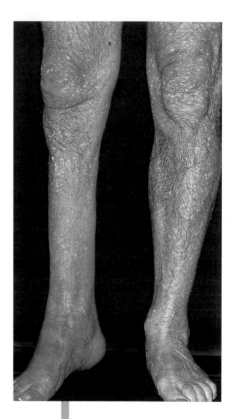

Legitimate uses of anabolic steroids

Anabolic steroids are prescribed by doctors to treat some medical conditions. Their main use is in the treatment of a few rare forms of severe anaemia. They may also be prescribed to reverse the effects of muscle wasting, which can be seen, for example, in people who are immobile for a long period after having major surgery, people who are suffering from malnutrition, or people with AIDS-related weight loss.

Muscle wasting

Steroids can help rebuild muscle in cases like this, where one leg has been immobile after an accident and its muscles have wasted.

The androgenic (sex hormone-like, or masculinizing) properties of steroids can be useful for treating males who cannot naturally produce enough testosterone. For patients like these, taking steroids can be helpful in speeding up delayed puberty or improving sexual function.

Anabolic steroid abuse

Non-medical use of anabolic steroids is commonly referred to as 'steroid misuse' or 'steroid abuse'. People who abuse anabolic steroids are often trying to boost their athletic performance or improve their physical appearance.

The anabolic steroids that are abused usually come in two forms: tablets that are taken orally (swallowed) or capsules containing liquids. The liquids have either an oily or watery appearance and are taken by injection, usually into the large muscles of the buttocks. Other less common preparations of anabolic steroids include patches, implants or sub-lingual pellets (tablets that are placed under the tongue and allowed to dissolve).

Abused drugs
Anabolic steroids are manufactured in many different forms.

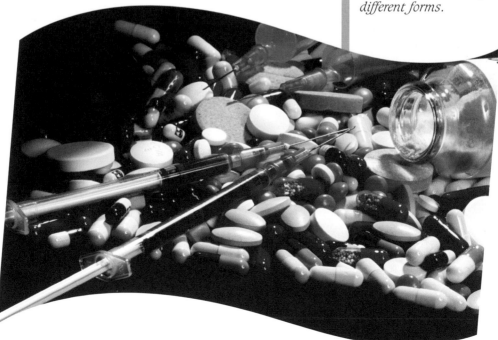

Slang terms for anabolic steroids include 'roids' and 'gear', or users may simply refer to them by the commercial trade names of the individual drugs. Commercial names vary from country to country, but may include: Stromba, Deca-Durabolin, Primobolan, Anavar, Winstrol, Anadrol, Dianabol and Sustanon 250. Sometimes veterinary anabolic steroids are sold to abusers too, commonly a brand called Equipoise that is designed for horses.

When someone is taking anabolic steroids for non-medical purposes, they usually take the drugs for a set number of weeks and then stop to allow their body to have a break for a few more weeks. This is known as 'cycling', and the break is sometimes called an 'off-cycle'. Most users recognize that taking the drugs has a toxic effect on the body, and that taking them for a long period of time is particularly harmful. They may also believe that taking the break makes the next batch of drugs more effective, although this has not been scientifically proven.

'Some guys in my class have been experimenting with combinations of steroids and weird supplements. You should hear them talk! They think they're being scientific, but it sounds like guess-work to me.' (Liam, aged 16)

If a single drug is being taken, the user may start off at a very low dosage, then increase the amount over the course of several days. When they reach a maximum or 'peak' dosage, they begin to reduce the amount they are taking, then tail this off to zero and take a break or 'off-cycle'. This practice is sometimes called 'pyramiding'.

Some anabolic steroid abusers take a number of different drugs at the same time, rather than keeping to one type of steroid. This way of taking drugs is known as 'stacking'. A 'stack' of drugs can include various different anabolic steroids, street drugs or sports supplements with drug-like actions, all in a variety of different combinations and dosages. Users may believe these combinations have specific benefits, such as helping them to train harder or longer at the gym, although the theories behind 'stacking' have not been properly proven to be either effective or safe.

Team pressure

Joe is 16 and plays American football for a successful youth team. It's a hard team to get into, and requires plenty of commitment for the training and the travel. For the last two seasons the team has been top of the league, beating all the others in the country. Past members of the team have gone on to good colleges and high-profile jobs.

The coach pushes them hard, and tries to get them to keep to a healthy lifestyle. He has also warned the lads in the team away from using steroids and other drugs, but Joe knows that at least three of his team-mates have used them before. They all feel that they are under pressure to keep up their current winning streak, and some of them are also complaining of feeling tired and worn out.

Joe understands why they have been tempted to take drugs, but he turned them down when they were offered to him. He says that he wants to find out exactly how far he can go with just his own hard work and natural talent. He is also worried about harmful side effects. Although his drug-using team-mates look healthy now, Joe wonders what kind of health problems they can expect if they keep taking the drugs for months or even years.

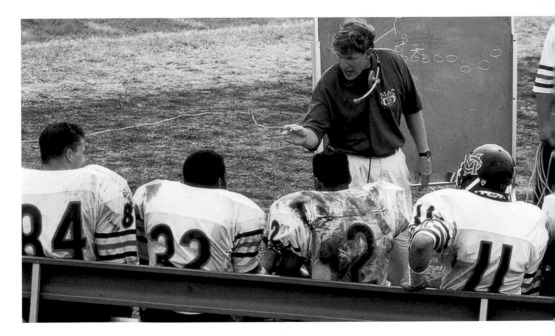

Anabolic steroids and the law

Under British law, anabolic steroids are treated as Class C drugs by the 1971 Misuse of Drugs Act. The Medicines Act classes them as 'Prescription Only' drugs, which can only legally be sold by a pharmacist who has been given a doctor's prescription. Since 1994 the maximum penalty for any other kind of supply is five years' imprisonment or an unlimited fine, or both.

Supply means selling drugs to other people (also called dealing) to make money, or simply giving them to someone without asking for any money. For example, a person who gives away two anabolic steroid tablets to a friend could be charged with supply. It is also illegal to possess anabolic steroids with 'intent to supply', but it is not illegal to possess small amounts for personal use.

Drug-like training aids from health food stores

Anabolic steroids are often taken in a 'stack' with a number of other drugs and drug-like supplements. The use of these supplements seems to have become more common, and in recent years the number of different products available has also increased. Some of the products mentioned on pages 15-17 are completely legal to use and are openly sold in health food stores, but others are now considered to be potentially dangerous and their legal status is under review in several countries.

There is more information about the possible side effects of some of these products in Chapter 3, along with

Training aids
Training aids are available from health food stores, but this does not mean that they are healthy. They may have the same dangerous side effects as anabolic steroids.

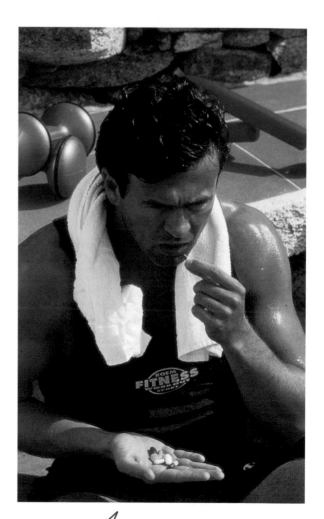

information about other substances that are sometimes added to 'stacks'. The category of 'drug-like training aids' does not include simpler nutritional supplements such as multivitamins or protein drinks.

Ephedrine

This is a stimulant (energy-increasing) substance extracted from a plant known as Ephedra or Ma Huang. The plant is sometimes used in oriental medicine as a tonic. Products containing Ephedra or Ma Huang are sold legally in the USA. In the UK, they are banned, although purified ephedrine is found legally in some decongestant tablets and nasal sprays.

Ephedrine increases the user's heart rate and sense of alertness. It gives a rush of energy, and is sometimes taken just before a workout to give the user the drive to work harder and push themselves further physically.

'I often take health supplements to give me more energy. If it's legal, then it's safe, surely?'
(Anita, aged 14)

There have been several reported cases of serious side effects, and this drug-like supplement has also been linked with a number of deaths. In spite of these warnings, ephedrine has been marketed as an ingredient of several different 'training aids', which also contain a number of other potentially harmful substances.

Caffeine

This naturally occurring stimulant substance is found in coffee, tea, chocolate and colas. Large amounts of purified caffeine are added to certain 'training aids' to give an energy boost before someone starts exercising, or the substance might be taken in the form of caffeine pills. Some 'training aids' mix caffeine with ephedrine. Caffeine is also found in several brands of painkillers and in cold and flu cures available from chemists.

Taking high doses of caffeine causes sleep disturbances and a feeling of jitteriness or irritability. Deaths from caffeine poisoning have also been reported occasionally, although the amount needed to kill an adult is a single dose of around 10 grammes, the equivalent of 100 strong cups of coffee.

Androstenedione ['andro']

Synthetic androstenedione and a similar substance called dehydroepiandrosterone (DHEA) are supplements that can be bought without a prescription in the USA. It is thought that once consumed, these substances may be converted into testosterone inside the body. (Both androstenedione and DHEA are produced naturally by the human body, in small amounts, and can be converted into both testosterone and the female sex hormone oestrogen.)

'Two of my friends have been stirring these powders into drinks before they go to the gym. I looked at the container but I have no idea what these ingredients are. Is it safe to take it?' (Bella, aged 14)

If 'andro' and DHEA supplements are converted into testosterone, it is likely that their negative side effects will be the same as those of anabolic steroids.

Nandrolone precursors

Some food supplements available as training aids are now thought to contain 'nandrolone precursors'. These are non-steroid substances that appear to be converted inside the body into an anabolic steroid called nandrolone, when the person who has eaten or drunk them also takes strenuous exercise. If these permitted chemicals are capable of being converted into nandrolone, then it is likely that they have the same health risks as the other anabolic steroids.

'It's big business, food supplements. Some of these shops are run by decent people who care about your health, but others will sell you anything to make money. It's hard to work out who the good guys are.' (Andrew, aged 18)

It is very difficult to tell whether a training aid contains nandrolone precursors, partly because labelling can be confusing and so many ingredients are added to the products. One study of nutritional supplements found that 15 per cent of them contained substances that could get a

A costly cold treatment

At the 2002 Winter Olympics in Salt Lake City, a drugs test found that skier Alain Baxter had taken a banned substance. He had to give up the medal he had won and was banned from competition for several months. After an appeal, it was agreed that Baxter had not deliberately taken the drug. It had entered his system from a nasal spray he had used to clear blocked sinuses.

sportsperson banned from competitions – so it is relatively easy to take banned substances by mistake.

There have been several cases of athletes who have tested positive for nandrolone and been thrown out of competitions, but who strongly deny ever knowingly taking the banned anabolic steroid. However they readily admit that they have consumed certain permitted training aids while they prepared for the competitions.

Risk warning

Anabolic steroids and supplements that have 'drug-like' effects all have a number of unwanted side effects. Some of these are minor or go away soon after the user stops taking the drug. Other side effects can be permanent or even life-threatening. The negative effects on women and teenagers are often the most extreme and long-lasting, but all users of these drugs should know that they are taking risks with their general health and wellbeing.

Becoming involved in drug-taking can also lead people into serious trouble with the law. A criminal record can affect a person's chances of gaining good employment for the rest of their life. A positive test for drugs usually ruins the promising career of any young athlete. Using anabolic steroids to gain an unfair advantage in a sport is also cheating, and gives the sport a bad image.

2 Patterns of use
Who uses steroids and why

People were taking substances to improve their performance in sport as long ago as the original Olympic Games in ancient Greece. Young athletes there were given special foods, such as sheep testicles, in the hope that these would help them to run faster. In the late nineteenth century, long-distance cyclists and competition swimmers reported using a wide variety of chemicals, including caffeine and nitroglycerine, in order to boost their stamina and chances of winning. These practices were frowned upon because they were potentially dangerous, and many people thought that taking drugs was cheating. Several cyclists taking the drugs collapsed during or after races, and a number of them died as a result.

In 1935, scientists in Amsterdam succeeded in isolating a chemical from bull testicles that they identified as testosterone. In the same year, another pair of researchers discovered that giving this extract of testosterone to dogs caused an increase in the muscle mass of these animals, under certain conditions. In the late 1930s, testosterone was being used to treat teenagers with hypogonadism, a medical condition where the testicles do not naturally produce enough testosterone. When this affects young men, there is not enough of the sex hormone to stimulate normal growth, or for the changes that happen at puberty.

Ancient Olympians
The sheep testicles eaten by athletes in ancient Greece may have provided them with extra testosterone.

Early steroid abuse in sport

It is thought that by the late 1940s a few Russian weightlifters had discovered testosterone and had secretly begun to use it because they believed it increased strength and muscle growth. Around the same time, doctors began treating patients with testosterone for conditions other than hypogonadism, such as muscle wasting and anaemia. They wished to avoid the androgenic (masculinizing) side effects of the drug when treating these illnesses, and so by the 1950s several new 'less androgenic' anabolic steroids had been developed.

Some weightlifters at the 1954 Olympics were thought to be abusing anabolic steroids, and in 1956 the steroid Methandrostenolone (Dianabol) was marketed widely in the USA, where it came to the attention of bodybuilders and strength athletes. This paved the way for more widespread abuse among some of the world-class high-strength athletes in the 1960s, even though many judges and competitors thought it was a dishonest way of gaining an advantage. Medical experts raised their concerns many times about the safety of non-medical steroid use, and in 1975 the International Olympic Committee finally banned the drugs, after accurate blood and urine tests became available for checking if people had been taking them. Several governments around the world made it illegal to traffick (transport and sell) anabolic steroids for non-medical purposes.

Seventies Olympians
The increasing abuse of steroids undermined the Olympic principle of fair competition.

By the mid-1970s, the use of anabolic steroids had spread beyond the Olympics to many other sports, partly because sportspeople believed that the drugs would allow them to recover more quickly after training. Drug regimes were made up by guesswork and passed on in secret by word of mouth. They were never based on scientific facts or proven to be safe. Routine drug testing was introduced in many sports, although it did not seem to deter some of the abusers, and many famous athletes failed the tests. Any Olympic athlete found to have taken anabolic steroids was banned from ever taking part in the Olympics again and stripped of any medals they had won.

In 1983, nineteen athletes were disqualified from the Pan-American Games for anabolic steroid abuse. After another round of disqualifications and a two-year investigation, the US federal grand jury charged 34 people with steroids trafficking in 1987, and former Olympic medal-winning athletes were among those fined and sentenced to prison. Since then, several promising sporting careers have been destroyed by positive 'doping' (drugs) tests.

Anabolic steroid abuse in sport today

Most people would agree that taking drugs such as anabolic steroids to gain an advantage is cheating, and there is no place for it in sport. In addition to the general health risks outlined in Chapter 3, sportspeople who use anabolic steroids have an increased chance of injury due to over-exerting themselves during training, and often lose the concentration and focus that are vital to success because the drugs have a negative effect on their mental state.

Golden moment?
At the 1988 Olympics in Seoul, South Korea, Ben Johnson set a new record winning the 100 metres sprint. But a drug test revealed he had taken anabolic steroids and he was stripped of his gold medal.

However, in spite of the risks to their health, reputations and careers, certain sport users still look for ways around the ban on steroid abuse in competitions. For example, they take new performance-enhancing drugs that are currently undetectable, or they consume chemicals that may mask the effects of the steroids. This may be because they have become obsessed with winning at any cost, rather than doing their personal best and winning fairly. Many athletes say that they are under enormous pressure to perform, whether this is pressure from family, coaches and sponsors, or pressure to gain sports scholarships and get into a good college.

Falsely accused

Tina was a successful sprinter and hoped to compete in the Olympic Games. She says that she never knowingly took anabolic steroids or other banned substances, but tested positive for them during a national athletics heat. She appealed against the decision, hoping that there had been a laboratory error, but when the tests were repeated, once again she was found to have taken steroids.

It was a serious setback to her career, and her personal life. Her sponsors cut off the funding that allowed her to train, she was banned from competing at national and international level, and friends and fellow athletes branded her a liar and a cheat. She spent two years trying to clear her name, but with little success. Eventually, her coach was accused of 'doping' two other girls in his team without their knowledge. He had been hiding oral steroids and other performance-enhancing drugs in food and drinks that were given to the athletes.

Tina decided that she'd been away from training so long that she would never regain her original level of fitness, so she decided to begin a business degree instead. Although she is happy with the way her life has turned out, she still wonders what it could have been like if she'd had the chance to go to the Olympics.

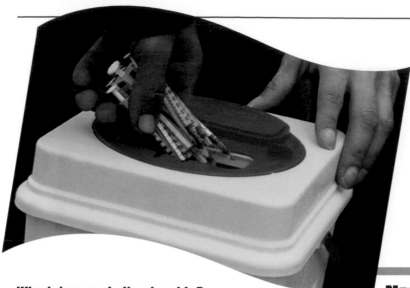

Who takes anabolic steroids?

There is no typical anabolic steroid abuser. The people who take these drugs come from rich and poor backgrounds, and are of all ages, races and nationalities. Males are more likely to abuse steroids than females, but there appears to be an increasing trend for young women to take these drugs.

In the UK, studies have estimated that up to 4 per cent of college students have tried anabolic steroids, half of them to 'enhance appearance' rather than improve athletic performance. Surprisingly, needle exchange programmes set up to deal with heroin addicts commonly report that around one third of their clients are anabolic steroid injectors, most of whom are bodybuilders. This suggests that steroid abuse is more widespread than previously thought in the UK, and that many bodybuilders are aware of the health risks of using shared or dirty needles.

Research presented at a British Medical Association conference in 2002 suggests that there are 45,000 British gym-goers who regularly use steroids, and many more who have tried them. Overall, it has been estimated that 5 to 9 per cent of gym users take anabolic steroids, but that figure may be as high as 20 to 40 per cent in particular gyms. Around a third of family doctors in the UK have encountered steroid abuse in one or more of their patients.

Needle exchange

Steroid abusers make up a large proportion of the people who return used needles in needle exchange programmes.

'I was watching the wrestling on TV and told my brother I'd like to give it a try when I was older. He said they were all taking anabolic steroids and covered in fake tan and makeup, they weren't really as cool as they looked. But they can't all be taking drugs, can they?'
(Sol, aged 14)

Strong and popular?

'I was shy and skinny, and wanted to be more like my loud, sporty classmates. I'd been bullied badly when I was younger, and figured that people wouldn't pick on me so much if I was bigger physically.

I began to train at home and gained some muscle using dumbbells, but soon I wanted to join a gym, to use more specialized equipment. I felt more confident fit, although I was still a bit shy. But no matter how much weight I gained, I never felt quite muscular enough. Eventually I met someone through the gym from whom I could buy anabolic steroids, and I thought this was the answer to all my problems.

After packing on some more muscle, I was so pleased with my body, you couldn't keep me away from the mirror. But I had a shock on holiday, when I stripped off down to my swimming trunks on the beach. A gang of teenagers went by and laughed, calling me a 'drug freak' and saying that my body looked disgusting. Maybe they didn't realize I could hear them, but I was shocked to think that some people found my appearance repulsive.

After that, I stopped taking steroids and spent less time lifting weights, and took up martial arts classes instead. They help you develop an inner strength. They've helped me feel more relaxed, and I know I would be able to defend myself if I was ever physically attacked. I've grown to like the new size and shape of my body, and think I'm healthier now, both mentally and physically.' (Dan)

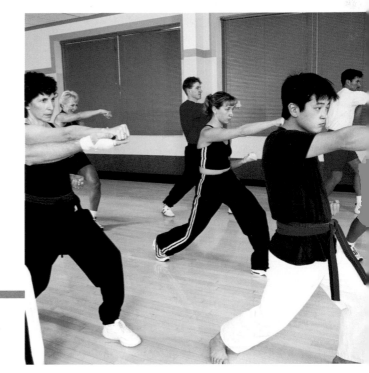

Martial arts class
Many people find that learning a martial art helps build their self-confidence.

3 Steroids and the body
The physical risks of anabolic steroids

There are many health risks associated with taking anabolic steroids. This chapter looks at the physical risks, and Chapter 4 explores the range of mental and emotional effects. Because these drugs are sold illegally, buyers are always in danger of receiving fake or contaminated products, which is the case with most street drugs too. Many people who abuse anabolic steroids do so by injecting them, and this has specific health risks.

'I could never inject myself. I can barely let a doctor near me with a needle! Injecting is dangerous, I know. But I heard that taking steroids as tablets is bad too, because it puts strain on your liver.'
(Vana, aged 16)

However the steroids are taken, they can permanently affect the growth of teenagers and the physical appearance of women, as both these groups are especially vulnerable to the unwanted side effects of the drugs. In addition, anabolic steroids can cause serious problems with vital organs such as the liver, heart and kidneys. They can also affect bones and joints, and cause a variety of other problems such as unhealthy skin and premature hair loss.

Veterinary and fake drugs

Many forms of anabolic steroids used by bodybuilders and athletes were originally intended for veterinary use, as a booster to help sick and injured animals to recover quickly. They were designed to be suited to the body size and metabolism of animals such as horses. The same drug can have different effects in different animals, so it is not right to assume that what works for horses is safe or effective for humans. Some of the people who abuse these preparations wrongly imagine that taking the drugs will help them to have muscles like those of a race horse, but this is not the case.

Some of the chemicals sold as 'steroids' are counterfeit (fakes) and could contain absolutely anything. Factories making fake steroid drugs have been found in Mexico, Eastern Europe and India. The manufacturer or seller is usually more interested in making a profit than in the buyer's health.

Counterfeit glass phials sold illegally as 'anabolic steroids' have been found to contain nothing but inactive substances such as water or vegetable oil. More disturbingly, they may contain high levels of bacterial contamination, or other deadly toxins. There is no way to tell exactly what is in them without sophisticated laboratory tests.

Dangers of injecting

Using needles is a very high-risk activity. Injecting steroids into the buttocks or other muscles carries most of the same risks as injecting other street drugs. Repeated injections into the same area over a long period of time can eventually lead to the formation of ugly scar tissue. A user may accidentally jab a needle into a nerve, causing damage that results in an unsightly and painful swelling which is difficult to get rid of. It is also possible to accidentally inject into a vein or artery, and this can cause gangrene (death of body tissues) or even be fatal.

Scars
People may inject anabolic steroids to improve their body image, but repeated injecting can result in ugly scars.

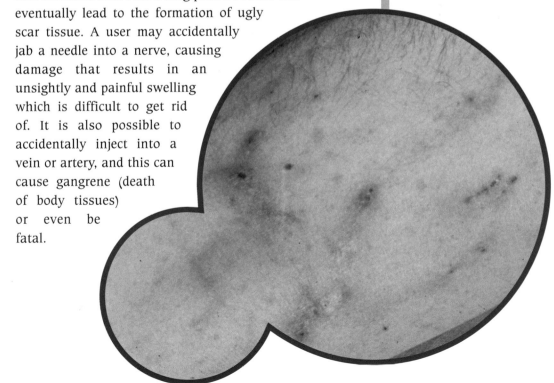

Because users find it hard to reach their buttock muscles, friends or training partners often inject one another. This sometimes means that they end up sharing needles and syringes. Just because a friend or acquaintance looks healthy, there is no guarantee that they are not carrying a potentially deadly virus such as HIV (the virus that causes AIDS) or hepatitis B or C. These viruses are spread by sharing needles. Dirty needles infected with bacteria can also cause life-threatening abscesses (painful and tense collections of pus) or blood poisoning.

How steroids can lead to stunted growth

During a normal, healthy puberty and adolescence, changes in the natural levels of hormones in the body cause a growth spurt – a rapid increase in height over a relatively short period of time. At the ends of each long bone, such as the femur (thigh bone) in the leg, there is an area called the epiphysis, which is slightly softer than the rest of the bone around it. The epiphysis is the place where most new bone structure is produced, making the biggest contribution to the final length of the limb. When the person has reached their maximum height, the sex hormones signal the bones to stop growing. (This final height is mostly determined by the height of the person's parents, general health and eating the right food.) The end of the growth period is caused by the epiphysis becoming hardened and making no more new bone.

Bone growth
At puberty, hormones stimulate the production of new bone at the epiphysis, resulting in a 'growth spurt'.

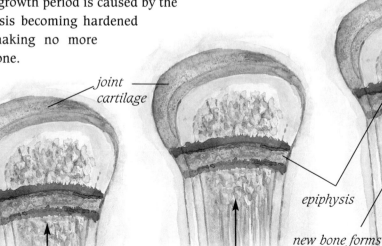

new bone hardens on this side

joint cartilage

epiphysis

new bone forms on this side

Large doses of illicit anabolic steroids during the teenage years can act like an incredibly high level of natural sex hormones, causing the ends of the bones to stop growing far too soon. The result of this is stunted growth, which is permanent. In other words, the person never reaches the maximum height they could have reached, and ends up much shorter.

'I really hate to see teenagers taking steroids because they can stunt your growth and cause all kinds of other problems.'
(Patrick, competition-level bodybuilder, aged 34)

More trouble with bones and joints

The rush of energy or aggression that steroids can give encourages some people to push their body too far when they are training. This can cause irreversible changes inside their joints, where bone starts to rub against bone, and the damage eventually leads to a condition known as osteoarthritis. Osteoarthritis is deformed, worn-down, painful and stiff joints and is a permanent condition. Sufferers may have joint pain for the rest of their lives, sometimes accompanied by loss of mobility.

The tendons and ligaments that support the joints can also be strained by training too hard, and so the joints are weakened. Some bodybuilders have ruptured tendons (completely tearing them away from the nearby bone) or torn muscles after training too hard. There have also been reports of steroid abusers tearing muscles or snapping tendons after very minor injuries.

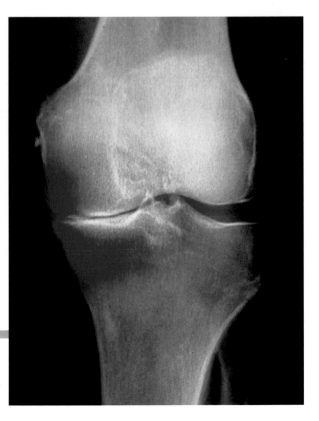

Osteoarthritis
This coloured x-ray shows loss of cartilage in the knee joint, causing bone to rub against bone.

Skin problems

Steroids act as hormones, which means that they deliver chemical messages to a number of different cells and tissues around the body. (See the sections on Hormones and Cell receptor sites on pages 8-9.) If a steroid molecule binds to a receptor site on the cell surface of an oil gland in the skin, this acts like a switch, speeding up the cell's functions. In the case of oil glands, this means that droplets of oil are pushed out onto the surface of the skin much more rapidly than before. Increased oil production can cause extremely greasy hair and skin, spots, worsening of existing acne and sometimes cysts.

High dosages of anabolic steroids can also cause bruising of the skin, stretch marks (which never completely go away), hives and other unattractive and itchy rashes.

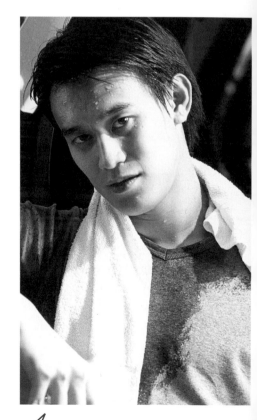

Steroids made his acne much worse

Mike had been using steroids for a few weeks when he noticed that his hair had become greasy and he had acne on his face, chest and back. As no over-the-counter acne remedies would work, Mike went to his doctor, thinking he needed some stronger medication.

The doctor said Mike's acne looked much worse than when he'd had it in his early teens, and so he'd need to do a full examination and some blood tests. He noticed that Mike had been working out heavily and asked if he had been using steroids – he pointed out that Mike wouldn't get into any trouble for telling the truth. Mike admitted the extent of his drug use, and the doctor explained that this was almost certainly what was causing the damage to his skin. Mike agreed to stay away from steroids and, after intensive antibiotic treatment, his skin started to improve. He says he wasn't tempted to take more steroids: there was no point having bigger muscles if he was going to be covered in acne all the time.

Why baldness happens

When testosterone has done its work in the body, enzymes break it down and a chemical called dihydrotestosterone (DHT) is made. In people of a certain genetic type, if DHT binds to receptor sites on the surface of their hair follicle cells, this signals the follicles to shrink. The hair will then start to grow thinner and shorter, and become less deeply rooted, and eventually bald patches start to show.

Male pattern baldness

Bald patches appear on the top of the head and around the front of the hairline. Follicle cells in these areas are the most sensitive to DHT, possibly because they have the largest number of DHT receptors.

Hair loss

Anabolic steroids can cause a form of premature balding in many young people. This specific type of hair loss is called 'male pattern baldness', and can happen severely in both men and women who use anabolic steroids for non-medical purposes. Certain people seem to be naturally more at risk of male pattern baldness than others; this is down to their genetic makeup and is especially likely if baldness runs in their family. People who might eventually naturally lose some hair in their fifties or sixties can put themselves at high risk of going bald in their teens and twenties if they abuse anabolic steroids.

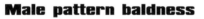

'My older brother used a lot of steroids last year. He wanted to look really buff and become a bodybuilder. The drugs made most of his hair fall out. He's tried everything to get it to grow back but nothing has worked.'
(Richard, aged 14)

Liver damage

The liver is a large and active organ. It is vital for removing toxins from the body and processing a wide range of chemicals and hormones. Steroid abuse has been linked to several forms of liver damage, and the steroids thought to place the greatest strain on this organ are those that are taken by mouth.

Anabolic steroids appear to cause damage to the cells in the liver, but fortunately the liver's activity returns to normal after the drug usage is stopped. Long-term, extra-heavy doses of steroids might also increase the risk of liver cancer and of a rare form of hepatitis (liver inflammation) where blood-filled sacs form inside the liver. These liver cancer tumours and sacs sometimes cause internal bleeding.

Hepatitis viruses can be spread by sharing dirty needles and can cause inflammation of the liver. Over time, this may lead to the

Organs at risk
Anabolic steroid abuse brings a risk of damage to the working of all these vital organs.

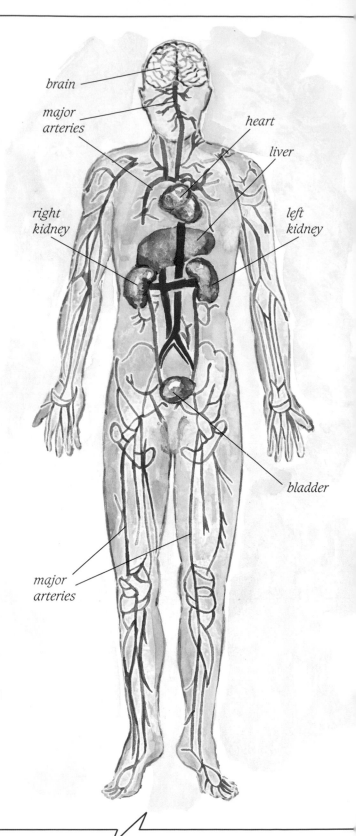

brain

major arteries

heart

liver

right kidney

left kidney

bladder

major arteries

liver becoming badly scarred (cirrhosis), and there is an increased risk of liver cancer. Hepatitis C is one type of virus that can be passed on by dirty needles, and can cause years of ill health, liver failure and even death. It is very difficult for doctors to treat, so prevention of new infections is the best way to stop the person-to-person spread of this disease.

Kidney problems

The kidneys are also very active organs, found in the pelvis and connected to the bladder. They help remove toxic chemicals from the body and carefully regulate levels of water and salt. This balance is vital for life.

Doctors have suspected for quite some time that long-term abuse of steroids has played a part in damaging the activity of the kidneys or causing kidney tumours in some people. Although many people who abuse anabolic steroids often refuse to admit that their drug-taking is harmful to their health, they often deliberately avoid alcohol because they believe that a combination of alcohol and steroids places an especially dangerous strain on the kidneys.

On dialysis
A kidney dialysis machine removes waste products from a patient's blood.

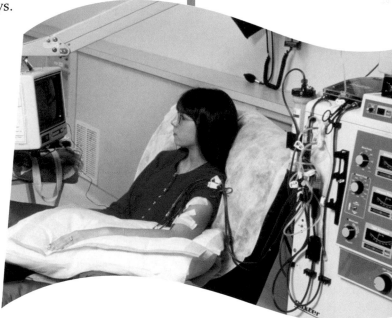

When a person's kidneys stop working properly, this is called kidney failure or renal failure. The person must have dialysis (using a machine to clean their blood) for the rest of their lives, or needs a kidney transplant; otherwise they will die. Many people who have kidney failure feel permanently tired and ill, and using a dialysis machine usually means spending many hours in hospital every week.

Heart and blood vessels

A healthy blood pressure is due partly to the force of the heart pumping blood around the body and partly to the resistance of the blood vessels. Abusing anabolic steroids both makes the heart work harder and affects the resistance of blood vessels by altering cholesterol levels.

High blood pressure (sometimes known as hypertension) can be caused when steroids encourage the body to retain too much water and the heart has to work harder to keep the extra fluid moving around the veins and arteries. High blood pressure can damage the delicate tissue that lines the arteries, as the changes in blood flow cause the artery walls to become narrow and weak.

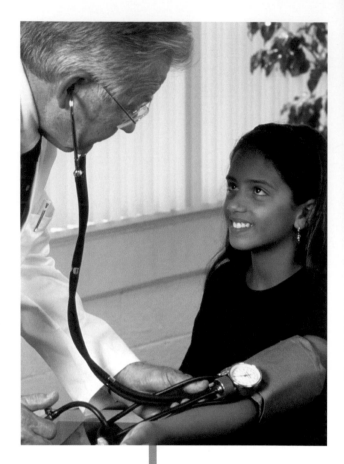

Blood pressure

Blood pressure is measured with a sphygmomanometer. A rubber cuff is placed around the arm and inflated until the pulse can no longer be heard. As the cuff is deflated the pulse is heard again. The first and second sounds give the blood pressure reading on the gauge.

Holding water

The commonest side effect seen in people who use anabolic steroids for non-medical reasons is fluid retention (oedema or 'holding water'). Up to half of all steroid abusers may suffer from this, where the body is not able to regulate its fluid levels properly and excess water ends up stored in body tissues. It gives rise to a 'puffy' or bloated appearance in the face, hands or ankles. Although the users may be trying to gain bigger, more defined muscles, the fluid actually makes muscles less visible.

Arteries

When fatty deposits build up on the insides of the arteries, there is less room for blood to flow through, and a clot may form.

blood flow through normal artery

Cholesterol and the arteries

When the lining of the arteries is healthy and smooth, blood can flow easily around the body. As people grow older, or if they eat a diet including a lot of unhealthy fatty foods, fatty deposits build up on the insides of the arteries, making it harder for the blood to flow through.

blood flow through artery with fatty deposits

Abuse of anabolic steroids stimulates the liver to increase the levels of LDL (low density lipoprotein) cholesterol in the blood. This form of cholesterol, also known as 'bad cholesterol', is the type that clogs up arteries, and is another major risk factor for heart disease and stroke. Steroid abuse also seems to lower the levels of HDL cholesterol ('good cholesterol') that would normally help to keep the arteries clear of fatty deposits.

formation of blood clot blocks the blood flow

If high blood pressure damages the arteries that feed the heart, the person may suffer heart disease such as angina (crushing chest pain) or even a heart attack (also called myocardial infarction) where part of the heart muscle dies because its blood supply has been cut off.

'I had to call an ambulance to my gym last week. Some stupid kid collapsed in the changing rooms after taking too many steroids. If I caught you using drugs here, I'd definitely throw you out.'
(Mac, gym-owner, aged 29)

If high blood pressure stretches the delicate and sensitive arteries that supply the brain, this can lead

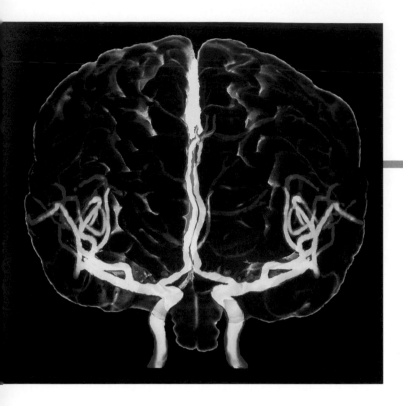

Healthy brain

This MRI scan shows healthy arteries delivering blood to the brain. If the blood supply to the brain is restricted, an area of brain tissue becomes starved and dies.

to severe headaches or even blackouts (loss of consciousness). Eventually these arteries may become weakened enough to cause a stroke, where the blood supply to part of the brain is cut off and an area of brain tissue dies. Strokes can result in permanent disability and are often fatal.

Colds, flu and general physical problems

Steroid users seem to catch colds and flu more frequently than most people. There may be swelling of lymph nodes (the 'glands' in the neck, armpits and groin) after taking the drugs. Many users complain of frequent nosebleeds or headaches too, and can suffer from sore throat, sore tongue and bad breath.

Effects on males

There are some side effects of taking anabolic steroids that are specific to boys and men. These are mostly caused by the androgenic (testosterone-like) actions of the substances.

Many male steroid users say that their libido (sex drive) is increased when they start a new course of the drugs. They sometimes find that their erections (where the penis becomes hard during sexual arousal) last longer than usual, and there can be the unwanted effect that erections happen at inappropriate times and will not go away. However, increased libido does not last.

'When my brother worked as a bouncer, he was injecting steroids and going to the gym five days a week. He used to joke about his balls shrinking, but I bet he was secretly embarrassed about it. I would be.'
(Ian, aged 13)

High doses of anabolic steroids eventually make the body shut down its own natural production of testosterone, so that libido then goes down drastically. Reduced natural testosterone can also make it difficult to get, or keep, an erection. Other unwanted side effects include reduced sperm production (temporary infertility) and shrinkage of the testicles.

When there are large amounts of testosterone-like substances in the body, they can be metabolized into other hormones. This process is called aromatization, and can lead to the production of oestrogen in males. This increased amount of female sex hormone may cause the growth of breast tissue beneath the man's nipples. This tissue remains under the skin after the person stops taking their course of steroids. The only way of getting rid of the unwanted growths is by having surgery.

'If you ever buy bodybuilding magazines, look at the pecs. Some guys are growing breast tissue because of the steroids. Some have strange scars around their nipples from the surgery to remove it.'
(James, aged 18)

Effects on females

Women's bodies do naturally produce tiny amounts of testosterone, which is needed for wellbeing. However, taking large doses of anabolic steroids (testosterone-like substances) can cause some very extreme changes. In females, most of these effects are irreversible.

- **Facial changes:** The skin becomes rougher, coarser and more oily, and delicate features can start to look more masculine rather than feminine. Facial hair begins to grow darker and thicker.

- **Body changes:** Sex hormones cause the tissues around the vocal cords (the larynx or voice box) to thicken, causing the voice to become permanently huskier and deeper. This process is similar to the natural breaking of a boy's voice at puberty. There may also be an irreversible increase in growth of body hair, and the breasts can shrink. Loss of breast tissue can only be corrected by surgery. In some women, another permanent change is that the clitoris may become enlarged.

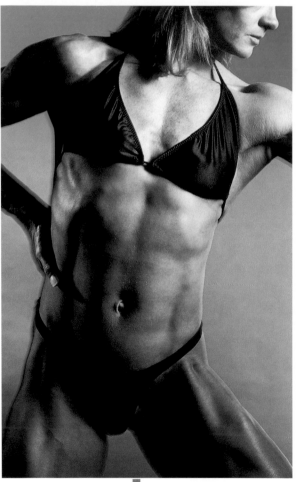

A new look
The unwanted effects of steroid abuse on a female body are usually irreversible.

- **Reproductive system changes:** Periods can become irregular, or may stop altogether. There is a risk that if a woman takes anabolic steroids when she is pregnant, a miscarriage or stillbirth is more likely. Anabolic steroids during pregnancy can also cause physical deformities in the baby.

Changes to the female physique, including muscle growth and loss of a 'feminine' appearance, often cause social stigma.

Facial hair nightmare

Maria trained hard as a swimmer from the age of ten, and began competing at county level in her early teens. She was one of the best swimmers in the county, but found it very hard to cope when she reached only third or fourth position in the most important races of the season. Her best efforts never felt quite good enough.

A team-mate convinced her that the winners had all been using illicit drugs and taking banned supplements to give themselves the edge. This helped him to persuade Maria to buy steroids from him. After a few weeks of injecting the drugs, her skin seemed less soft. Then she noticed dark, thick hairs growing on her upper lip and chin. She was shocked because her team-mate had told her that these changes would not happen with the drugs.

Maria spoke to her doctor and was devastated to find out that the changes to her skin were permanent. A long, expensive and painful course of electrolysis was needed to get rid of the facial hair. Although she does not think of herself as a vain person, Maria has been very upset by the changes in her appearance.

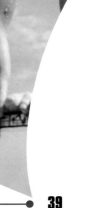

Other drugs taken in 'stacks'

Many of the following drugs are abused along with anabolic steroids. The practice of 'stacking' (taking more than one drug at the same time) increases the risk of unwanted side effects because each of the following compounds has its own risks.

- **Nalbuphine hydrochloride** (Nubaine/Nubain): This drug is an analgesic (painkiller) that some people inject before a workout. It prevents them feeling the pain of over-exertion, and this makes serious injuries much more likely. Nalbuphine also has a mood-altering effect, and is opiate-based like drugs such as morphine and heroin. This substance is highly addictive, and even most steroid abusers describe it as 'far too dangerous to use' or 'a junkie's drug'.

- **Clenbuterol hydrochloride:** Clenbuterol is medically prescribed for the treatment of asthma, but it is sometimes abused because some people think it can burn off fat and slow down the process where the body breaks down protein. Side effects include tremors (shaking), high blood pressure, difficulty sleeping, and headaches.

- **Diuretics:** These drugs stimulate the flow of urine, and remove fluids from the body. Bodybuilders sometimes take them before shows to counteract the fluid-retaining side effects of steroids, and to make their muscles appear larger. Unfortunately, strong diuretics also remove vital minerals and salts such as potassium along with the fluid, and this can cause cramping and collapse.

- **Erythropoietin** ('EPO'): This is an injectable synthetic hormone that stimulates the body to make more red blood cells. This allows the blood to carry more oxygen, theoretically increasing a person's ability to exercise, although it has never been shown to improve athletic performance. More cells in the blood make it thicker, and this increases the risk of life-threatening blood clots in deep veins or the lungs, heart attacks and strokes.

4 Steroids and the mind
The mental and emotional risks

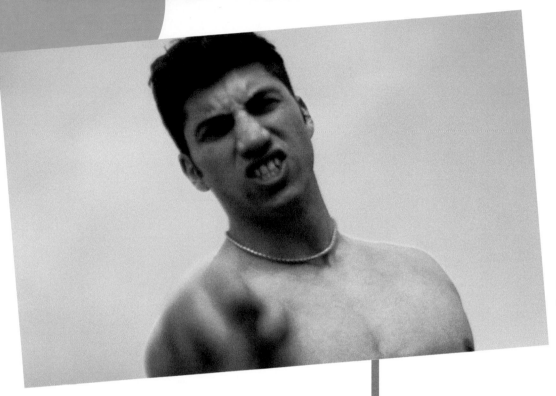

Anabolic steroids can affect the way you think or feel. They do not always cause the extreme and unpredictable violence (also known as 'roid rage') that is reported in the tabloid press. The psychological changes can sometimes be quite mild, or even pleasant, which encourages some users to take more.

The effects of anabolic steroid abuse can include feelings of energy or motivation, but these drugs can also cause irritability, aggression, anxiety and sleep disturbances. In a few people, steroids have been linked to violence, depression and paranoia – a mental condition where the person is severely suspicious or mistakenly thinks that they are being persecuted.

Roid rage
Sudden loss of temper for no good reason is one of the emotional effects of steroid abuse.

Energy and motivation

In some people who take anabolic steroids there can be a sense of self-confidence and attractiveness and a feeling of increased motivation and energy. Users who go to the gym or do sports say that they are able to train harder and longer because of this feeling of motivation. Some people find these feelings are so pleasant that they want to keep taking more and more of the drugs, even if their health suffers as a result.

'For a few weeks I felt invincible, and the life and soul of every party. Later, after I came off the steroids, people told me how full of myself I'd become, and how much they hated the way I'd been acting.'
(Ellie, aged 17)

The feelings of confidence can become dangerous when they make someone feel as if they are all-powerful and indestructible, when of course they are not. This has been called 'The Superman Syndrome', and is probably due to a combination of the mood-altering effect of the drugs and the increased physical strength and muscle mass that follow heavy training.

Over-confidence may lead to people training so much that they damage their bodies, or to them taking stupid risks with their safety, such as driving dangerously or putting themselves in situations where they might be attacked. Over-confidence can also make a person appear arrogant or 'pig-headed', and may cause problems with family, friends and people at work or college.

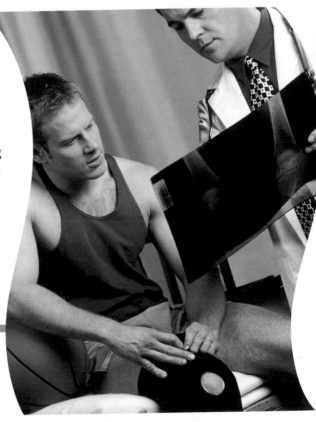

Over the top
The extra energy that steroids give can lead abusers to exercise so hard that they injure themselves.

Irritability and aggression

Many anabolic steroid users admit that the drugs make them feel more irritable, snappy or aggressive sometimes, and often say these feelings are worse if they are taking higher dosages. They may say that the feelings of aggression can be used to help them train harder when they are exercising. They also point out that feeling more aggressive does not necessarily translate into mindless violence, because most people who take anabolic steroids are able to exercise self-control over their moods and behaviour.

The person who is taking the drugs may deny that they are behaving in an anti-social way, and might not even realize how bad-tempered their actions have been. However, the steroid abuser's family or friends may be much more aware of the snappiness and mood swings.

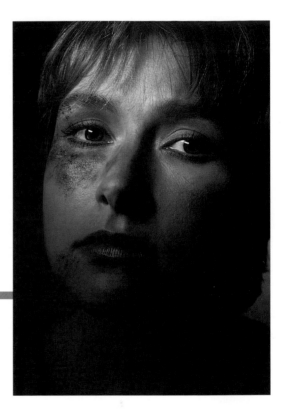

Domestic violence
An abuser's lack of self-control can sometimes have tragic results.

Violence

Non-medical use of anabolic steroids has been linked with domestic violence, rape and other sexual assault, attempted murder and aggravated robbery. There have been several court cases where the legal defence has suggested that steroid abuse left a person in such a disturbed mental state that they were not responsible for their actions.

Roid rage
'Roid rage' is a slang term for a sudden loss of temper and extreme violence, and although it's not that common, it does happen to a few steroid abusers. The person often completely over-reacts to something minor that would not bother most people.

People who take anabolic steroids often say that those who behave aggressively or violently on these drugs are naturally aggressive or violent people. They seem to think that steroids bring out the worst in people who are 'bad' already. Many researchers disagree with this, and think that steroids can have this effect even on people who are easy-going and have no history of violence. They say that it's not possible to predict who will become aggressive.

I just snapped

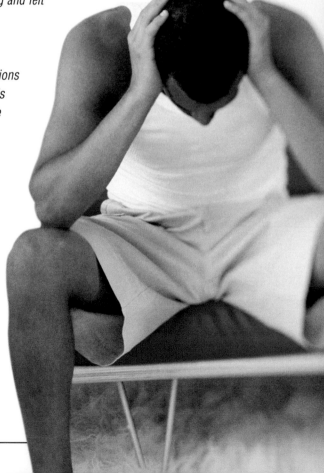

Anthony had always considered himself a go-getter and very competitive. He was not someone who got into fights. He was popular at work and had a long-term girlfriend. He attended the gym regularly, and after trying a short course of one type of steroid, Anthony felt that his looks had improved, although he was having trouble sleeping and felt irritable fairly often.

Ignoring the side effects, he took a combination of several steroid preparations without taking a break, or 'off-cycle'. His moods worsened, and one afternoon he had an argument with his manager and ended up throwing a chair across the office. That evening his girlfriend challenged him about his drug-taking. The discussion quickly escalated into screaming and shouting, and Anthony lashed out, punching her.

She ended the relationship and will no longer have anything to do with him. Anthony bitterly regrets what happened, and says she made the right decision. He says he takes full responsibility for his actions because he chose to take the drugs in the first place.

Anxiety and sleep problems

Some steroid users say they get insomnia (difficulty sleeping). This may mean difficulty getting to sleep at night, having nightmares that wake them up, sleeping less deeply than usual, or waking up early and not being able to get back to sleep.

Although some people who abuse anabolic steroids say that the drugs help them to be more motivated, many others say that they have difficulty concentrating when on the drugs. This can cause a variety of problems in everyday life, especially in situations that need full concentration, such as exams, sporting competitions, driving a car or riding a bike in traffic.

The need to concentrate

Lack of concentration in an important exam can have far-reaching consequences.

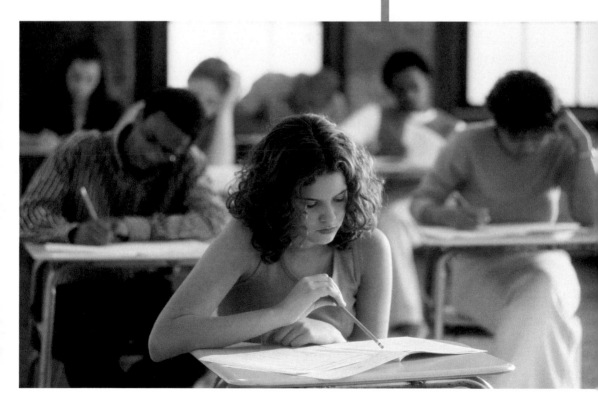

Steroid users often say that they have higher levels of anxiety and stress. There may be unpredictable feelings of fear, agitation or jitteriness, or even strong sensations of panic.

Paranoia and other mental illness

There may be a tendency for anabolic steroids to make underlying mental health and personality problems worse. Anyone with a history of mental illness should completely avoid anabolic steroids. Some people can become paranoid when on steroids, which means that they feel deeply suspicious of others, or afraid of being harmed, or think that they are being persecuted.

Someone who is paranoid cannot understand that they are not really in danger, and they may act in strange or harmful ways because they wrongly believe that they need to defend themselves. In extreme cases, sufferers may have to be hospitalized for their own and others' safety.

Depression

Some users say that steroids make them feel very down and miserable. If these feelings are strong and last for a long time, the person can fall into a state of depression, and they may start to feel that life is not worth living. The feelings of depression can last for as long as it takes the body to clear out all traces of the drug. This can be up to a year with some types of steroid.

In the 'off-cycle', when the user stops taking steroids for a period to 'rest' the body, there may be feelings of depression, tiredness or powerlessness. A few people say that they experience deep distress at the loss of some of the muscle that had been gained.

'It sounds stupid now, but I took some steroid tablets because I was going on a beach holiday and wanted to wear a bikini. After four weeks I was so depressed I could hardly work. The moods went on for months.'
(Ashley, aged 16)

Psychological dependency

Some people who take anabolic steroids end up feeling that they cannot function properly in everyday life without them. This is known as becoming psychologically dependent on, or psychologically addicted to, the drugs. People become dependent like this for different reasons.

They might start to rely on the feelings of energy and motivation they get from anabolic steroids, becoming hooked on the feelings of power or thinking that they are unable to motivate themselves with willpower alone. They might start to think that they cannot perform properly in sport without the drugs. People who have abused steroids to cope with feelings of being 'not physically good enough', 'not strong enough' or 'unattractive' may find it difficult to cope when the drugs are out of their system and their body starts returning to a more natural size and shape.

People who become dependent on anabolic steroids continue to abuse them even though their health is obviously suffering. They carry on taking the drugs even in spite of the likelihood that they will be thrown out of college, get into trouble with the police, be dropped from the sports team or asked to leave home.

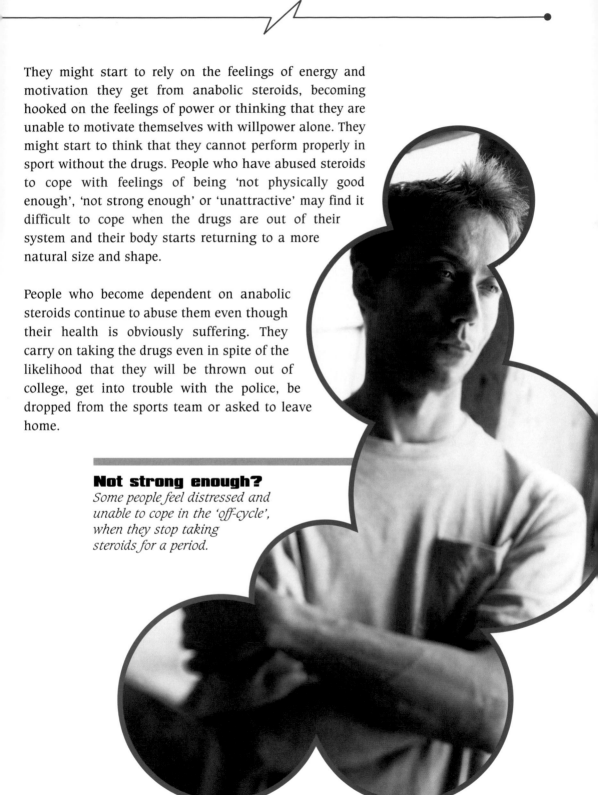

Not strong enough?
Some people feel distressed and unable to cope in the 'off-cycle', when they stop taking steroids for a period.

Signs of developing dependency

- Losing friends or finding family relationships strained because of your drug use.
- Taking higher and higher doses of anabolic steroids.
- Continuing to take the drugs after a 'cycle' has finished.
- Stealing money, or borrowing money that you never intend to pay back, to pay for drugs.
- Missing work, college or school because of the side effects of the drugs.
- Continuing to take drugs and train, even though you are not well or have an injury that needs resting.
- Mixing anabolic steroids with illegal drugs such as amphetamines ('speed') or injectable painkillers to make yourself train even harder.
- Feelings of paranoia or irritability while taking anabolic steroids.
- Lying about the extent of your drug use, or covering it up.
- Feeling down, powerless or depressed after coming off anabolic steroids, and then taking more drugs to avoid these feelings.
- Wanting to give up, but not feeling able to do so.
- Continuing to abuse steroids even after others have given strong warnings of the consequences, such as losing a job, ending a relationship or being thrown off a team.
- Becoming obsessed about where the next batch of drugs is coming from.

'I hated the way that I'd go from feeling like a superhero to feeling lifeless and worthless on an off-cycle. I started to wonder what it would be like if I got rid of the off-cycle altogether.'
(Marshall, aged 16)

'If you'd told me then that I was wrecking my body, health, studies and relationships, maybe a part of me would have believed you – but I would never have admitted it to anyone, not even myself.'
(Lara, aged 18)

Admitting I was hooked

'I'd been weight-training for three years before I started taking anabolic steroids. After a few weeks I was very pleased with the changes in my physique. I almost felt like a Greek god! But friends and relatives commented that I had become obsessed with my appearance. I felt much more attractive when I was highly muscular and taking steroids, and hated being reminded about how skinny I once was.

When I took a break at the end of the first cycle of steroids, I lost some of the muscle I'd gained. I felt as if I was shrinking and becoming ugly again. I couldn't cope with the way I felt. I began to take anabolic steroids without an off-cycle, even though I knew it was dangerous. Deep down I wanted to stop, but just couldn't face the weight loss that would follow, and I was hooked on the feeling of energy that I got from the drugs.

After a few months, and several injuries from over-training, I decided that my body couldn't take the strain much longer. I began to attend a drug dependency project, came off the steroids completely, and had a long course of counselling to help come to terms with my poor body image. Admitting that I had a problem with anabolic steroids was one of the hardest things I've ever had to do, but it was worth owning up to it.'
(Sanjeev, aged 21)

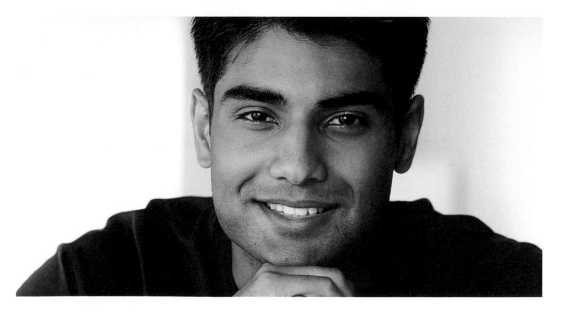

5 Giving up steroids
Helping yourself or others

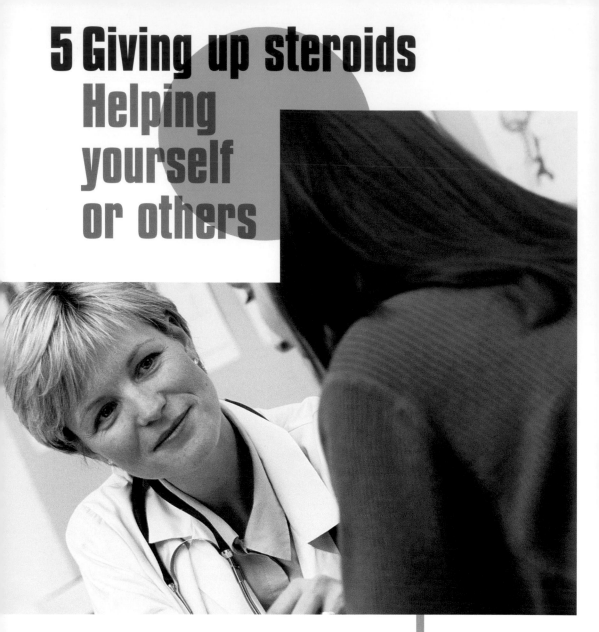

This chapter looks at what it's like to come off steroids, and what help is available for people who want to stop taking them. It also considers ways of addressing some of the underlying problems that may lead people into abusing these drugs in the first place.

You may be concerned about a friend, partner or relative who is or might be abusing anabolic steroids. This chapter also gives advice on what to do in this situation. Emergency information is included on pages 58-59, explaining what to do if someone becomes tense and aggressive, or passes out or collapses.

Seeking help
Admitting to yourself that you have a problem with taking steroids, is an important first step. Then your doctor will be able to help you give up the drugs.

Giving up steroids

Many people who take anabolic steroids find that they can give them up without any serious problems, but some users find that stopping taking the drugs has unpleasant effects. The effects are mostly short-term, and pass in a few days or weeks. They include feelings of tiredness, lack of energy and sometimes depression. If untreated, feelings of depression may sometimes last up to one year.

'I felt washed out for a month or so after giving up, and was tempted to go back to steroids. I had headaches and felt very down at times, although my family were supportive. I'm proud that I saw it through.' (Chris, aged 17)

There may also be restlessness, disturbed sleep and reduced appetite. A few people report symptoms such as headaches, muscle and joint pains, chills (shivering) and nausea (feeling sick). Prolonged use of anabolic steroids leads to the body shutting down its own natural production of testosterone, so there can be a long period where someone has a lack of libido (sex drive) and other sexual problems.

Once the use of anabolic steroids has stopped, there is a loss of some of the muscle that has been gained. People with low self-esteem or poor body image often find this loss of size extremely distressing, and feel tempted to take more drugs to make themselves feel better. If a user is convinced that they cannot perform well without anabolic steroids, they may feel a strong desire to continue using the drugs, rather than fail to meet their own (or someone else's) high standards.

'My GP suggested cutting down slowly rather than stopping suddenly, but explained that I might still have mood swings and other temporary problems.' (Terry, aged 19)

The family doctor can help and support someone trying to give up anabolic steroids. Doctors can give information about the drugs, provide a thorough physical check-up, and refer people to drug agencies or for counselling. They can provide treatment for any unpleasant effects of giving up steroids. Doctors must keep anything they are told confidential, and cannot report a young person to their parents or the police. However, if the young person is being pressured into taking the drugs, for example by a sports coach, the doctor must report this, as it is a form of abuse.

Some people may not want to talk to their family doctor about their steroid abuse. They may prefer to ring a drugs helpline instead. These helplines are completely confidential. They can give out advice about the drugs, or refer callers to local drop-in centres or nearby drug counselling services. Several useful helplines are listed on page 62.

'My counsellor showed me that there were lots of alternatives to taking drugs every time I needed a boost. I feel more able to talk through problems, rather than losing my temper or giving up and walking away.'
(Billy, aged 19)

Better ways of problem-solving

An important part of coming off anabolic steroids is to understand what was making you take them. Then you may be able to find other ways of dealing with the issue, which are healthier and more likely to succeed.

For some people, taking the drugs and excessive exercise are ways of ignoring or trying to alter unpleasant feelings, but this is likely to backfire in the long run. A better way of coping with thoughts and emotions that are worrying you and getting you down is to find someone to talk to whom you trust. This could be a friend, a relative, your family doctor, a teacher or a school nurse. You might be more comfortable confiding in someone you don't already know, such as a professional counsellor.

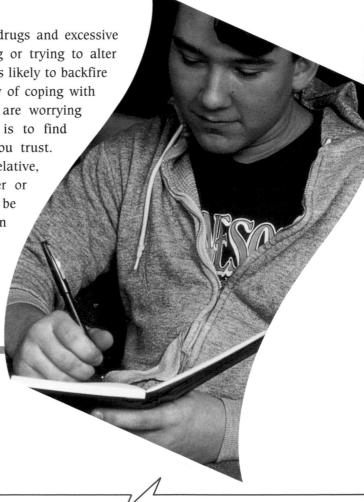

Writing it down
If you don't feel you can talk to someone about your problems, it may help to write about them.

Sometimes, people take anabolic steroids in the belief that they will make them feel stronger and more confident. One healthier way of building self-confidence is to sign up for a course of assertiveness training. This shows people how to stand up for themselves in a positive way, without the need to behave aggressively. People who feel weak or vulnerable to attack without anabolic steroids could also try self-defence classes or learn a martial art.

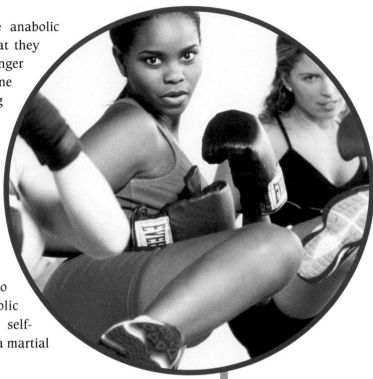

Coping with pressure and perfectionism

Many people start taking steroids because they think they need them in order to win at sports, or to boost their performance in other ways. Putting this kind of pressure on yourself, or constantly striving to be perfect, can be very unhealthy. To take some of this pressure off, concentrate on performing to the best of your ability, not on being 'number one' or getting 100 per cent every time. Set yourself realistic targets, such as running a race in a set period of time, rather than beating someone else.

Self-defence
Learning kick-boxing is a healthy way of overcoming lack of confidence, as well as keeping fit.

If you don't reach the target that you've set for yourself, do not tell yourself that you are a failure. It's OK to make mistakes, and many useful things can be learned from these experiences. What seems to be a 'failure' can turn into a real success. For example, it was a failed experiment that led the scientist Alexander Fleming to discover the antibiotic penicillin. If his original experiment had not gone wrong, he may not have discovered this important drug, which has saved many thousands of lives.

If coaches, friends or family are putting too much pressure on you to do well, thank them for their support but point out that you are already trying as hard as you can. You may have to decide to avoid certain people if they are putting you under an unreasonable amount of pressure. If you can't avoid them, make sure you spend time with other people who can help you keep the situation in perspective.

Remember that human beings are not machines, and they are not supposed to be perfect! A healthy, happy life is all about balance.

Healthier ways to feel fit and attractive

Very many people who abuse anabolic steroids do so in a quest to achieve a different look, which they believe will make them more attractive. However, what makes a person attractive to another is not something skin-deep. Almost always, when people find someone attractive, they say this is because of something like the person's happy smile or sense of humour. These things have nothing to do with the size of a person's muscles, or how thin their thighs might be. People of all colours, shapes and sizes can be described as attractive.

Winning looks
A friendly smile is more likely to win someone over than having a particular appearance.

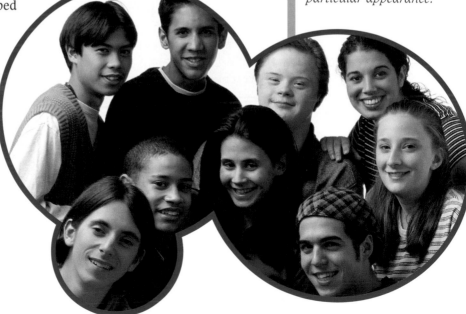

Make a list of all your good qualities that have nothing to do with appearance: this could be anything from being a great friend, being good at sports or music, or doing well with grades at school. Looks don't count at all with these sorts of things. If you find yourself obsessing about your looks from time to time, get this list out and have another look at it. You could even pin it to your mirror or carry it around in your wallet so that you can see it every day.

'My best friend is kind, but the best thing is she's completely honest. If I start slipping back into obsessing about my appearance, she gives me a reality check. She reminds me of all the good things going for me.'
(Cath, aged 18)

Concentrate on being healthy, rather than forcing a particular appearance on yourself. Eat a balanced diet, get enough sleep and look after your hair, skin and teeth. Regular moderate exercise is the best way to tone up, and will give you a genuine healthy glow and an energy boost. It's not a 'quick fix', but you should see the benefits within a few weeks.

Are you really too flabby or not muscly enough? Ask a few level-headed people whom you know and trust. If your appearance makes you desperately unhappy, but everyone who knows you says you look fine, think about asking your doctor to refer you to a counsellor who can help you gain a more positive body image.

Is someone you know abusing steroids?

There are several signs that suggest that someone may be abusing anabolic steroids. However, some of these can also be part of normal teenage physical changes and behaviour, so you should not automatically assume that someone who looks or behaves in these ways must be taking drugs.

- Increased acne, especially on the back, or greasier hair and skin.
- Bruising more easily, or getting stretch marks.
- Hives or other strange rashes, or a flushed face.
- Head-hair loss in males and females.
- Rapid weight gain over a few weeks or months.
- Puffy appearance to the face, hands or ankles.

TO31121

- Sore throat, sore tongue or bad breath.
- More frequent headaches or nosebleeds than usual.
- Growth of breast tissue in males, or shrinking breast size in females.
- Growth of facial and chest hair in females.
- Strained relationships with friends and family.
- Over-confidence or increased hostility or aggression.
- Sudden unexplainable feelings of frustration or anxiety.
- Difficulty sleeping, or increased restlessness.

Helping a friend

If you know that a friend is taking anabolic steroids, you may want to encourage them to stop and find help with giving up the drugs. So long as your friend is not being aggressive or irritable, talk to them and show concern about their use of anabolic steroids. Try not to start an argument; just say that you are worried about them, and explain why.

Do not do anything that will make it easier for your friend to carry on abusing steroids. Don't lend them money to buy more. Don't be persuaded to buy or hide their drugs for them, or cover for them if they make themselves ill or behave badly towards others.

'Thinking I could be a model, I tried silly crash diets and high doses of steroids. Nobody told me to stop taking the drugs. Perhaps they were scared of me as I was acting crazily. I wish they had, though.'
(Deanna, aged 15)

Make sure that you look after yourself properly too. It is difficult to be supportive if you are an emotional mess yourself. Talk to someone if it is stressful, and do not put up with verbal abuse or violence. No matter how much you want your friend to give up, remember that this is their responsibility, not yours. If they really don't want to stop abusing anabolic steroids, there may be very little you can do to help them.

If you are worried that they are putting themselves in serious danger, and they have refused to listen to you, you may have to decide to tell a responsible adult. It's understandable that you would be scared about ruining your friendship, but you might be helping in the long run.

Some friendly advice

Matt and Darren have known each other since they were five. They trained together at the local gym. Darren got interested in bodybuilding, and started injecting anabolic steroids. Matt was more relaxed about the way he looked, and didn't want to take drugs. Over a few weeks, Matt noticed that Darren's personality and behaviour were changing for the worse. He had become arrogant and bad-tempered, and wasn't even keeping up with his training at the gym.

Matt says he couldn't ignore these changes any longer and took Darren to one side for a chat. He told Darren that he thought he was damaging his body and relationships, and was getting nothing positive out of taking the drugs. He also explained what it felt like to watch an old friend do that to himself and the people around him.

Matt admits he was surprised when Darren agreed with him, but puts it down to the way he put his opinions across, and the fact that they are old friends who trust one another and are very honest. Darren had already decided that he was not going to inject any more drugs, but was glad of the moral support, and says it helped him to avoid the temptation of taking more.

He also thinks that everyone should be more aware of the number of young people who are abusing steroids, and of the wide range of risks that they are taking.

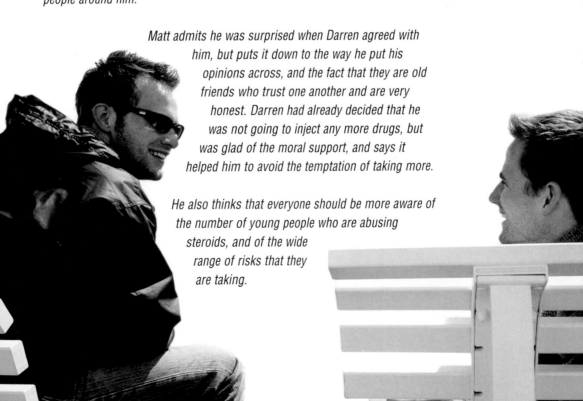

What to do if someone is anxious or agitated

If you find someone in an anxious or aggressive state, they might be under the influence of alcohol, street drugs, anabolic steroids, solvents or a mixture of all of these.

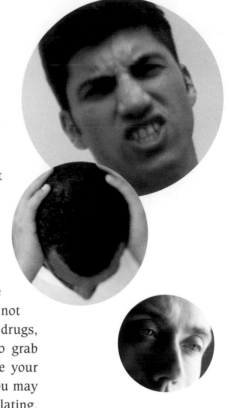

- Follow your instincts. If you have the slightest suspicion that the person may become violent, get out of there fast and call the police. Do not put yourself at risk. Running away is not a sign of weakness, and you should not be ashamed of doing so.

- Although this is a frightening situation, be careful not to show your feelings of panic. Do not become angry or shout at the person for taking drugs, even if they become unreasonable. Try not to grab them, lean over them, point at them or shake your finger. By not reacting in any of these ways, you may help to prevent an aggressive incident from escalating.

- If you are sure that the person is anxious but definitely not being violent, try to help them. Speak softly, get them to sit down somewhere quiet, and show them how to breathe slowly. Tell them gently that you will look after them until they are feeling better, to help reassure them.

- Do not give them coffee or any other drinks containing caffeine, such as tea or cola. These may make them more agitated or irritable, and can speed up the action of any drugs that are in their body.

- You may want to call an ambulance or doctor to be on the safe side. Collect up anything that appears to be connected to the incident and show it to the doctor or paramedics. This could be pills, glass capsules, powders, lighter fuel cans, glue, syringes or other suspicious items.

'I've seen guys freak out at my gym, getting all stressed and paranoid, not enough sleep. And I've seen a couple just black out after workouts – not sure what they were on. Nobody really knew what to do, it was scary.' (Richard, aged 17)

Emergency: what to do when someone is unconscious

If you find someone unconscious:

- ⚙ Call an ambulance immediately. Stay as calm as possible.
- ⚙ Gently try to wake the person, but do not shake them hard.
- ⚙ Check that they are still breathing by looking at the rise and fall of their chest or listening to the area around the nose and mouth. If they are not breathing, be prepared to do CPR (mouth-to-mouth resuscitation) if you have first aid training.
- ⚙ If the person remains unconscious but is still breathing, check their mouth for obstructions such as vomit. Quickly scoop out obstructions with your fingers. Loosen tight clothing to allow the person to breathe more easily.
- ⚙ Turn them on their side and put them into the recovery position. If they are sick in this position, there is less risk of them choking on their vomit.
- ⚙ If possible, make sure that the person is not left alone while you wait for the ambulance to arrive. Check from time to time that they are still breathing.
- ⚙ Collect up anything that appears to be connected to the incident and show it to the ambulance team. This could be pills, glass capsules, powders, syringes or other suspicious items.

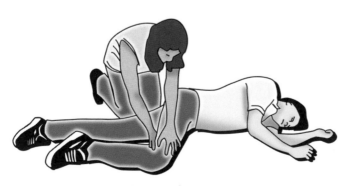

Recovery position

If someone is very drowsy or unconscious, you should put them into the recovery position. Lie them on their left side, with their right arm and right leg bent. This means that if they vomit, there is less risk of them choking on it.

Glossary

addicted emotionally or physically dependent on a substance or behaviour to get through everyday life, and feeling unable to give it up.

anabolic having the effect of stimulating the building up of molecules. The effect of anabolic steroids is to build up extra protein inside muscle cells.

anabolic steroids a group of man-made drugs that act like androgens, or male sex hormones.

anaemia a condition where there are not enough red cells in the blood, or not enough of the oxygen-carrying compound called haemoglobin. It is unusual for it to need treatment with steroids.

androgenic having the effect of the male sex hormones. These are the hormones that stimulate changes in males during puberty, causing growth of facial hair, or deepening of the voice, for example.

cardiac arrest the sudden stopping of the heart, which is often fatal.

cholesterol a fatty substance found in all human tissues and in the blood. High levels of one form of cholesterol have been linked to heart disease. The body can process cholesterol molecules to make steroids.

CPR cardio-pulmonary resuscitation. This first-aid technique may save the life of a person who is not breathing and whose heart has stopped beating. Also called 'mouth-to-mouth' resuscitation.

cravings unpleasant and intense desires or longing for a substance, especially felt when someone is addicted to it and is trying to give it up.

cycling a slang term for taking anabolic steroids for a few weeks, then not taking them for a few weeks, before starting to take them again.

cysts abnormal sacs or blister-like pouches in or on the body, containing fluid or semi-solid material.

dependency psychological or physical reliance on a substance, such as steroids or street drugs, usually with strong cravings.

doping giving drugs such as anabolic steroids to athletes and other sportspeople to give them an unfair advantage.

enzymes a group of complex protein molecules that assist in biochemical reactions.

hives a skin condition with itching and raised red or white patches, often caused by an allergy. Also called urticaria or nettle rash.

hormone a chemical substance that's released into the bloodstream and carried to certain cells where it attaches and causes changes in their metabolism.

hypogonadism a rare condition where young men do not produce enough male sex hormones, and their puberty and growth are delayed.

irritable quickly irritated, or easily annoyed.

libido — another name for a person's sex drive.

masculinizing — having the effect of making someone's appearance more 'manly'. Testosterone has a masculinizing effect on the hair on the face, making it grow thicker and darker.

metabolism — all of the chemical processes that take place inside a living organism. It includes growth, production of energy and breaking down of waste products.

nausea — the sensations that occur before someone vomits. Also described as 'feeling sick'.

oestrogen — one of the main female sex hormones, which plays a major role in regulating the menstrual cycle and changes that happen in the female body during puberty.

off-cycle — slang term for the break that is sometimes taken between courses of anabolic steroids.

peer pressure — pressure to behave in the same way as other people in the same social group, such as classmates or friends. There is often a fear of being unpopular or abandoned by friends, which can make it very difficult for an insecure person to stand up for themselves.

receptor — a highly specialized area on the surface of a cell, to which only one kind of molecule (for example, a steroid) can attach. Once this molecule has attached to the receptor, it acts like a switch, telling the cell to behave in a particular way.

self-esteem — a feeling of self-respect and liking yourself, feeling generally good about yourself.

skeletal muscle — the muscles on the outside of the body which are used during exercise. Not to be confused with the smooth muscle that's found inside arteries and the gut.

stacking — slang term for taking several drugs at the same time, often including more than one kind of anabolic steroid.

steroids — a large group of naturally occurring molecules that have a characteristic ring structure of four carbon atoms. The majority of them have important actions inside the body, such as the sex hormones.

stretch marks — red marks that appear in the skin after it has been stretched by rapid muscle growth or weight gain. The marks eventually fade to a slightly silvery colour.

testosterone — the most powerful of the male sex hormones, made in the testicles. Women also produce tiny amounts in their adrenal glands, found just above the kidneys.

toxin — a substance that is poisonous, harmful, or deadly.

veterinary drug — a drug that is designed to be used on animals, not humans.

Resources

United Kingdom Sports Council (UK Sport)

UK Sport are responsible for 'doping control' (drug-testing of UK sports competitors) and can give out plenty of information about anabolic steroids, banned supplements and other performance-enhancing drugs. Comprehensive 'doping' information can be found on their website.

Telephone: 020 7211 5100
www.uksport.gov.uk

National Drugs Helpline

This organization offers free and confidential advice about any drugs issue, including anabolic steroids, whether callers are looking for information, counselling or just a chat. It will try to help anyone who is having personal drug problems, and can give callers information about services that are available in their local area. Lines are open 24 hours a day. The website contains news and factsheets, and a confidential e-mail service for asking the experts questions about drugs.

Telephone: 0800 77 66 00
www.ndh.org.uk

DrugScope

This is a leading UK drugs charity and centre of expertise on drugs. It aims to provide balanced and up-to-date drug information to professionals and the public, and has a detailed factsheet about anabolic steroids on its website. There is also a searchable database of drug treatment and help services in England.

Telephone: 020 7928 1211
www.drugscope.org.uk

NHS Direct

This service provides information about anabolic steroid abuse as part of an online self-help information section. Includes statistics, dangers, and help for users and parents.

Telephone: 0845 46 47 (open 24 hours a day)
www.nhsdirect.nhs.uk

Disclaimer
The website addresses (URLs) included in this book were valid at the time of going to press. However, because of the nature of the internet, it is possible that some addresses may have changed, or sites may have changed or closed down since publication. While the author and the publishers regret any inconvenience this may cause readers, no responsibility for any such changes can be accepted by either the author or the publishers.

Index